POWER

OF

CO-ENZYME

Q 10

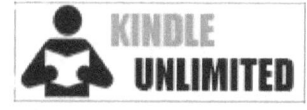

HEALTH SUPPLEMENT THAT COULD SAVE YOUR LIFE

Prem Chhatwani

Power of Co-enzyme Q 10

This publication is part of a Health Series of publications Vol. 6.

Copyright © 2015

Prem Chhatwani
Pjan International,
Inc.

negligence, accident, or any other
cause.

Preface

Over the years I had lot of interest in Alternate Therapies, including Homoeopathic medicines and Herbal and Ayurvedic treatments for various diseases.

At age 28 I got hit by Asthma. My Dad had Asthma and his younger brother (my uncle) had Asthma as well. My grandmother, father side, also had suffered from Asthma.

So I kind of inherited the disease but at a later age than as a child.

My Mom had heart problems but she actually died of Cancer in her late fifties.

With family history like that, I did not know what to expect in my older years. At age of around 50, with slightly high Cholesterol (230-240) and still using inhalers like Albuterol Sulfate and Cortisone (Prednisone) pills very frequently for my Asthma, I ran across some books and publications that opened my mind to try alternate remedies.

1) I started drinking Magnetized water every day as there were no side effects or interaction with my drugs for Asthma. One thing I must say Asthma patients should drink more water. Keep the body hydrated. The benefits of drinking magnetized water are realized very slowly but it also helps heart and lungs. It basically removes deposits from arteries and air passages in the lungs. Mind you, western medicine does not recognize this. Benefits of magnetized water would be another kindle book. If interested check this link but not required at all. http://www.amazon.com/dp/B007IO7DN8 Or simply email me at pjan86@gmail.com for a free report on this.

By Age 60 I was completely free from Asthma. Now I cannot prove Magnetized water did it. You the reader decide and investigate and be the judge. Main stream medical practitioners will make a fun of this. I got off my inhalers and Prednisone Cortisone pills which by the way affect bone density. I slowly improved my bone density with exercise, Calcium and Vitamin D.

2) I investigated Chelation Therapy. I found a certified Doctor, M.D. then in our small town in Ohio (USA). She was certified to do the procedure of administering by IV EDTA **(Ethylene Diamine Tetra Acetic acid) compound, approved by FDA for lead toxicity**. I could see her clinic full of patients hooked up IV rigs on wheels, reading books or working on their paper work. It was sight to be seen.

I decided to take two treatments a week, for six weeks. I never did consult my primary physician. I felt safe taking the treatment as a precaution to avoid heart problems in the future due to family history. I also had personal interest to see how it feels so that I can tell others my own experience. Once again I cannot recommend anything. There are several books on the subject. You can also read my Kindle book here: **http://tinyurl.com/n7r7ge6**

The best part now is that at age 77 I have no Asthma and my heart is healthy but I do take small dose of prescribed medicine for cholesterol to keep it under control. I do consume red meat, fish and drink red wine. I am seriously considering taking additional few Chelation treatments to help clean up my arteries as a precaution. I will consult an approved doctor trained and certified by ACAM for Chelation.

Let us now get back to main topic of this book "Co-Enzyme Q 10".

Table of Contents

1. A message from Dr. Crandall

Can CoQ10 Save Your Heart?

Dear Friend,

Hi, my name is Dr. Chauncey Crandall and I am a practicing interventional cardiologist, chief of the Cardiovascular Preventive Medicine Program at the Palm Beach Cardiovascular Clinic.

You already know how important the role of CoQ10 is to maintaining optimal cardiac health. Virtually every cell in your body contains CoQ10, which is concentrated in the mitochondria. Heart cells have approximately 5,000 mitochondria each, more than any other cells. In addition, CoQ10 is a strong antioxidant, which can help prevent premature aging and free E2554radical damage.

Today, numerous trials indicate CoQ10's unique ability to support heart health and function. Clinical studies on CoQ10 suggest that it can promote optimal heart function and normal blood pressure levels. Our bodies produce CoQ10 naturally, but unfortunately, our CoQ10 level declines with age. By the time you reach your 40s, your body's CoQ10 level may have dropped by as much as 30%. Taking statins drugs may also accelerate the loss of CoQ10 in your body.

2. Facts about Coenzyme Q 10

In addition to support heart health and to lower blood pressure by normalizing the body's a sodium/potassium ratio, it is interesting to note Coenzyme Q10 has positive effect on kidney functions as well.

A randomized, double-blind placebo-controlled study found that administering 60 mg of Coenzyme Q10, three times daily reduced the frequency of kidney dialysis after four weeks.

Creatinine and blood urea nitrogen levels were significantly reduced, and there was a marked increase in creatinine clearance and urine output.

Dosage: The "magic number" used in the vast majority of the research is 200 mg. Studies show that 200 mg daily from a CoQ10 supplement keeps your arteries relaxed and flexible, allowing blood to move freely through them, especially if you are over 50 years old.

Cardiologists often call CoQ10 the "miracle nutrient" because it fuels your cellular power plants. This is especially important for your heart—a muscle that requires huge amounts of oxygen and energy to function. Plus, CoQ10 acts as a potent antioxidant—hunting and destroying free radicals that can damage your heart health and overall well-being.

Medicines for high cholesterol (statins) and medicines that lower blood sugar cause a decrease of CoQ10 levels.

3. Is CoQ10 safe?

Taking 100 mg a day or more of CoQ10 has caused mild insomnia in some people. Research has detected elevated levels of liver enzymes in people taking doses of 300 mg per day for long periods of time. Liver toxicity has not been reported.

Other reported side effects include rashes, nausea, upper abdominal abdominal pain, and dizziness, sensitivity to light, irritability, headache, heartburn, and fatigue.

When using dietary supplements, keep in mind the following:

- Like conventional medicines, dietary supplements may cause side effects, trigger allergic reactions, or interact with prescription and nonprescription medicines or other supplements you might be taking. A side effect or interaction with another medicine or supplement may make other health conditions worse. Always tell your doctor or pharmacist about all dietary supplements you are taking.

- The way dietary supplements are manufactured may not be standardized. Because of this, how well they work or any side effects they cause may differ among brands or even within different lots of the same brand. The form of supplement that you buy in health food or grocery stores may not be the same as the form used in research.

- Other than for vitamins and minerals, the long-term effects of most dietary supplements are not known.

Watch this U-Tube video by Dr. Ray Sahelian, M.D.

CoQ10 benefit, side effects, coenzyme Q10 dosage, 30, 50, 60, 100 mg
https://www.youtube.com/watch?v=0kh-sCvmQvg

4. Ubiquinone Vs Ubiquinol

CoQ10 is a nutrient that is said to have profound effects on our levels of energy, stamina, organ health, and immune system functionality. CoQ10 comes in two forms: Ubiquinone and Ubiquinol. Ubiquinone (also known as Ubidecarenon) is more common and widely known because it is the form most commonly sold commercially. Ubiquinone is the completely oxidized form of CoQ10. When taken, this supplement is actually metabolized within our bodies where it becomes Ubiquinol. Regular insolubilized Ubiquinone does not dissolve in water and only poorly dissolves in fat. Therefore, regular insolubilized Ubiquinone has poor absorption.

Ubiquinol on the other hand is the strong, antioxidant form of CoQ10 which neutralizes free radicals and decreases cellular damage. Ubiquinone does not have this antioxidant effect. Ubiquinol supplements are in a form that has already been reduced to being a strong antioxidant. Ubiquinol is both water and fat soluble, so it provides superior absorption compared to regular insolubilized Ubiquinone. When taken directly in this format it works more quickly and can be delivered in lower concentrations without worry that it is not being metabolized.

The problem arises with aging in many people. The ability of the body to metabolize is reduced significantly over time and many older folks will find it is difficult for the body to break down Ubiquinone into Ubiquinol. Therefore, although it will come at a greater cost, taking Ubiquinol after the age of 40 is a good idea.

Individuals over the age of 30 typically begin to see deterioration in the heart, lungs and liver even when sustaining a healthy lifestyle. That's why it's important to understand the level at which your body functions and metabolizes food and supplements, so that you can make the appropriate choice between Ubiquinone and

Ubiquinol.

Primary dietary sources of CoQ10 include oily fish (such as salmon and tuna), organ meats (such as liver), and whole grains. Most people get enough CoQ10 through a balanced diet, but supplements may help people with particular health conditions or those taking cholesterol lowering statin medications, which wipe out CoQ10 from the body. Often those taking cholesterol lowering statin drugs like Lipitor, Zocor, Mevacor, Pravachol and Crestor have depleted levels of CoQ10. Adding Ubiquinol helps replenish missing CoQ10, sustaining the levels necessary to promote optimal heart health.

Ubiquinol is relatively new and more expensive to produce - so when the supplement contains Ubiquinol, the manufacturer is quick to point it out. When purchasing CoQ10, if the bottle does not mention which form it is, Ubiquinone or Ubiquinol, it is usually Ubiquinone as that is the cheaper of the two forms.

According to Dr. Sinatra's book about
Cariovascular Disease (available through
Amazon) you'll find that it's vitally important
to get a CoQ10 supplement that is
ABSORBED by the cardiovascular system so
that it can be dispersed through the tissues of
the body and into the cells for energy
utilization.

Well, run this test? Simply fill a glass with
about 8 oz. of warm water, then snip open the
end of a CoQ10 capsule and squeeze into a
puddle on top of the water. Come back in about
20 minutes and see if your CoQ10 is still
puddled. If it's still puddled together, don't buy
that brand again. ABSORBABLE CoQ10 will
disperse through the water and some may even
sink in ribbons to the bottom of the glass. I did
this test on some CoQ10 bought at Costco--IT
FAILED. Other CoQ10 recommended by my
doctor & bought at a health food store:
FAILED. Swanson's CoQ10? Passed the test! -
--AND-- it is a LOT less expensive & easy to
buy through Amazon.
Plus, I can also tell it is working because I can
definitely tell a difference as it helps improve

my energy level and mental sharpness--highly recommended!

Adding DHLA (The reduced concentrated form of Alpha Lipoic Acid) to CoQ10 increases its effect in addition it increases the effect of vitamin C and E.

When you add DHLA, you flood your cells with tremendous free-radicle fighting power.

I am over 70, I take 240 mg of R-Lipoic acid first thing in the morning. R-Lipoic acid is superior to Alpha Lipoic acid. Then I take 200 mg of Ubiquinol with breakfast or lunch...

Please check with your health advisor for proper dosage and guidance as to when to take it.

Note: Unfortunately main stream doctors do not advise well on health supplements as they are trained to promote prescription drugs.

Watch this informative U-Tube video here:

https://www.youtube.com/watch?v=JCr1EEdN mck

Testimonials collected from different sites:

I am 54 years old and I have gradually been getting more and more fatigued to the point where this year, it was a chore just to get out of bed. When I did, I spent most of the day lying on the couch. My legs were extremely fatigued just getting up and walking to the kitchen or bathroom. I tried all kinds of vitamins including B12, a B complex and D3. Nothing seemed to help. Went to my doctor and had blood tests done for thyroid, liver and kidney function and several other things. The results couldn't have been more NORMAL, yet, I was still feeling this chronic and debilitating fatigue!

Several weeks ago, I went on hormones and felt MUCH better, but was still not 100 percent myself.

I took a tablet of CoQ10 yesterday about 4pm and then again at 9pm. I woke up this morning almost my old self! I took the dog out and was able to walk a mile and a half in the park and my legs are barely tired!

I would highly recommend this to ANYONE who is experiencing symptoms of extreme fatigue and your doctor cannot find anything wrong with you and no amount, or type, of vitamins helps!

P.S. Make sure you eat a meal when you take CoQ10. The product information I read when researching the web sites that CoQ10 works much better when taken with a meal. It has something to do with the delivery method and being able to get into your system better when digestion is going on.

Additional Reviews

Reviewer: hootowl6087, 55-64 Female on Treatment for 10 years or more (Consumer)

Comment:
Been taking 200mg daily for over ten years. No longer get head colds, sciatica/back pain. Blood pressure is normal. Hoping it helps to keep heart healthy. People say I don't look my age....60 years.

ByChardon April 7, 2015

I was always fatigued and I was getting sick constantly, my body ached and even my skin and complexion looked awful. My physician told me to start taking Coq10. In less than a month, I felt great, the fatigue was gone, body aches gone and skin improved.

By Gem Dreameron November 11, 2013

I've never taken CoQ10 before and didn't really think I would see any results, however, after the first few days, I noticed a few changes. I noticed my energy level was higher and my concentration was better. After about a week taking the CoQ10, I took my blood pressure and thought the reading was a mistake. I took it again the next day and it was the same, the top number was down 10 points. I was shocked and elated. I told my Dad about it and he's now taking it. He said he noticed the same results, higher energy level, and better concentration. After two weeks, he took his blood pressure and it was down as well. I won't say if this product will work for you, but it definitely worked for me. Give it a try and see for yourself.

6. Resources

1) EDTA: This Four letter word may save your life
http://www.amazon.com/dp/B00GHC88BI

2) Herbs for Health and Healing
http://www.amazon.com/dp/B0080UVQUU

3) Pain Treatment
http://www.amazon.com/dp/B007IO7DN8

4) How to Prevent and Reverse Heart Diseases
http://www.amazon.com/dp/B00B4CQ3GS

5) Amazing Glutathione
http://www.amazon.com/dp/B00XWTX742

6) Power of Co-Enzyme Q 10

http://www.amazon.com/gp/product/B00ZRUBIZE?

Note: Please do read my above book #5.

It goes well with this book.

Amazing Glutathione. It is the protector and detoxifier of your body.

It is brief and to the point. Here is table of contents for your information.

1. **Introduction**

Your first line of defense against toxins, radiation, heavy metals, oxidative stress and accelerated aging. Glutathione helps protect

2. **What is glutathione**

Glutathione is a substance produced naturally by the liver. It is also found in fruits, vegetables, and meats.

3. **Benefits of glutathione**

Increasing your Glutathione level will naturally increase your energy, detoxify your body and significantly strengthen your immune system.

4. **How to improve GSH levels**

Glutathione taken orally is NOT well absorbed across the GI tract.

5. **Glutathione enhancing supplements**

We highlight a few of the most potent glutathione enhancing supplements and precursors

6. <u>How to take glutathione</u>

Orally or by Patch or by intravenously?

7. <u>Testimonials</u>

This will make a believer out of you!

8. <u>Glutathione, side effects and risks</u>

Some side effects may occur that usually do not need medical attention.

9. <u>Resources</u>